Dickson D. Despommier, Daniel O. Griffin, Robert W. Gwadz, Peter J. Hotez, Charles A. Knirsch

Clinical Appendix
for Parasitic Diseases
Seventh Edition

see full text of Parasitic Diseases Seventh Edition for references

Parasites Without Borders, Inc. NY

The organization and numbering of the sections of the clinical appendix is based on the full text of the seventh edition of Parasitic Diseases.

Dickson D. Despommier, Ph.D. Professor Emeritus of Public Health (Parasitology) and Microbiology, The Joseph L. Mailman School of Public Health, Columbia University in the City of New York 10032, Adjunct Professor, Fordham University

Daniel O. Griffin, M.D., Ph.D. CTropMed® ISTM CTH© Department of Medicine-Division of Infectious Diseases, Department of Biochemistry and Molecular Biophysics, Columbia University Vagelos College of Physicians and Surgeons, Columbia University Irving Medical Center New York, New York, NY 10032, ProHealth Care, Plainview, NY 11803.

Robert W. Gwadz, Ph.D. Captain USPHS (ret), Visiting Professor, Collegium Medicum, The Jagiellonian University, Krakow, Poland, Fellow of the Hebrew University of Jerusalem, Fellow of the Ain Shams University, Cairo, Egypt, Chevalier of the Nation, Republic of Mali

Peter J. Hotez, M.D., Ph.D., FASTMH, FAAP, Dean, National School of Tropical Medicine, Professor, Pediatrics and Molecular Virology & Microbiology, Baylor College of Medicine, Texas Children's Hospital Endowed Chair of Tropical Pediatrics, Co-Director, Texas Children's Hospital Center for Vaccine Development, Baker Institute Fellow in Disease and Poverty, Rice University, University Professor, Baylor University, former United States Science Envoy

Charles A. Knirsch, M.D., M.P.H. Founding Director of Parasites Without Borders, Inc.

Cover Design: Daniel O. Griffin (*Trichuris trichiura* adult male)

Page layout and design: Daniel O. Griffin

Editor: Angharad (Harrie) Bickle, Ph.D, PGCE.

Library of Congress Cataloguing-in-Publication Data

    p. cm.

    ISBN: ############ (PDF version)
    ISBN :########### (Kindle version)
    ISBN:9781098590482 (KDP)

    1. Parasitic diseases / Dickson D. Despommier, Daniel O. Griffin, Robert W. Gwadz, Peter J. Hotez, Charles A. Knirsch.
    IV. Title. Clinical Appendix for Parasitic Diseases Seventh Edition
    ©

Printed on paper made of pulp from trees harvested in managed forests.

© 2019 Parasites Without Borders.

All rights reserved. This work may not be translated or copied in whole or in part without the written permission of Parasites Without Borders (www.parasiteswithoutborders.com) except for small portions quoted in reviews or academic works. Any other use (electronic information storage, retrieval, or adaptation, computer software, or by similar or dissimilar methodology) is strictly prohibited. Our use of names, trade names, or trademarks in Parasitic Diseases 7th ed., even if they are not identified as such, must not be interpreted to mean that such names, as defined by the Trade Marks and Merchandise Marks Act, may therefore be used by anyone else. Neither the authors nor the publisher accept legal responsibility for any errors or omissions that may be made. The publisher makes no warranty regarding the material contained herein.

Contents

IV. The Protozoa
  1. *Giardia lamblia* — 1
  3. Cutaneous Leishmaniasis — 1-2
      Leishmania (L.) major
      Leishmania (L.) tropica
      Leishmania (L.) mexicana
  4. Mucocutaneous Leishmaniasis — 2-3
      Leishmania (V.) braziliensis
  5. Visceral Leishmaniasis — 3-4
      Leishmania (L.) donovani
      Leishmania (L.) infantum
      Leishmania (L.) infantum chagasi
  6. African Trypanosomiasis — 4-5
      Trypanosoma brucei rhodesiense
      Trypanosoma brucei gambiense
  7. American Trypanosomiasis — 5-6
      Trypanosoma cruzi
  8. *Trichomonas vaginalis* — 6
  9. The Malarias — 6-8
      Plasmodium falciparum
      Plasmodium vivax
      Plasmodium ovale
      Plasmodium malariae
      Plasmodium knowlesi
  10. *Cryptosporidium parvum* — 8
  11. *Toxoplasma gondii* — 8-9
  12. *Entamoeba histolytica* — 9
  13. *Balantidium coli* — 10
  14. Other Protozoa of Medical Importance — 10-13
      Babesia spp.
      Cystoisospora belli
      Cyclospora cayetanensis
      Naeglaria fowleri
      Acanthamoeba spp.
      Balamuthia mandrillaris
      Blastocystis hominis
      Dientamoeba fragilis
  15. Non-pathogenic Protozoa — 14
      Commensal Flagellates
      Commensal amoebae

V. The Nematodes

16. *Enterobius vermicularis*	14
17. *Trichuris trichiura*	14
18. *Ascaris lumbricoides*	15
19. The Hookworms	15
Necator americanus	
Ancylostoma duodenale	
Ancylostoma ceylanicum	
20. *Strongyloides stercoralis*	16
21. *Trichinella spiralis*	16-17
22. Lymphatic Filariae	17
Wuchereria bancrofti	
Brugia malayi	
23. *Onchocerca volvulus*	18
24. *Loa loa*	18-19
25. *Dracunculus medinensis*	19-20
26. Other Nematodes of Medical Importance	20-23
Capillaria hepatica	
Capillaria philippinensis	
Dirofilaria immitis	
Mansonella ozzardi	
Mansonella perstans	
Mansonella streptocerca	
Oesophagostomum bifurcum	
Ternidens diminutus	
27. Aberrant Nematode Infections	23-25
Cutaneous Larva Migrans	
Visceral Larva Migrans	

VI. The Cestodes

28. *Taenia saginata*	26
29. *Taenia solium*	26-27
30. *Diphyllobothrium latum*	28
31. Other Tapeworms of Medical Importance	28-29
Hymenolepis nana	
Hymenolepis diminuta	
Dipylidium caninum	
32. Juvenile Tapeworm infections of Humans	29-31
Echinococcus granulosus	
Echinococcus multilocularis	

  Mesocestoides spp.
  Spirometra spp.
  Taenia spp. (other than *saginata* and *solium*)

VII. The Trematodes

33. The Schistosomes   31-32
  Schistosoma mansoni
  Schistosoma japonicum
  Schistosoma haematobium
  Schistosoma mekongi
  Schistosoma intercalatum

34. *Clonorchis sinensis* and *Opisthorchis* spp.   32-33
35. *Fasciola hepatica*   33
36. *Paragonimus westermani*   33-34
37. Other Trematodes of Medical Importance   34-35
  Fasciolopsis buski
  Echinostoma spp.
  Heterophyes heterophyes
  Metagonimus yokogawai
  Nanophyetes salmincola

VIII. The Arthropods

38. The Insects   35-36
39. The Arachnids   37
40. Other Arthropods of Medical Importance   -

Exposures   38

Diagnostic and Laboratory Abnormalities   39

Symptoms   40

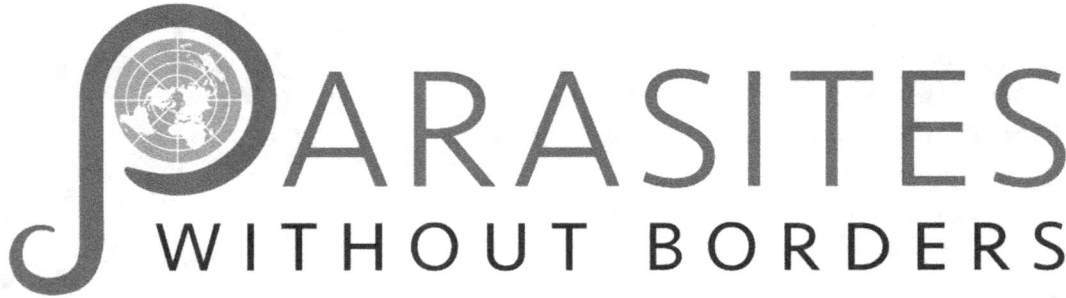

Parasites Without Borders was founded as a direct response to the question: "What can I do to help eliminate human suffering due to parasitic infections?" For us the choice was easy; more and better education for all those in a position to apply medical knowledge directly to populations in need of relief from the burden of parasitic diseases. The directors have a lifetime of experience in teaching parasitic diseases to students of medicine, both within the U.S.A. and abroad. Our mission statement is clear; we want to help bring the latest medical and basic biological information to every clinician and student throughout the world.

http://www.parasiteswithoutborders.com

Clinical Appendix

1. *Giardia lamblia*

Exposure Required:
Oral ingestion of cysts in fecally contaminated water or food

Clinical Disease:
- Asymptomatic
- Acute diarrhea, chronic diarrhea, foul smelling diarrhea, floating stools, flatulence, nausea, rarely fever, epigastric pain, weight loss, fatigue

Diagnosis:
- Stool ova and parasites (microscopic examination of stool)
- Antigen capture-ELISA from stool sample
- NAAT

Treatment:
- **Preferred drug options:**
    - Metronidazole 250 mg PO TID x 7-days
    - Tinidazole 2 g PO x1
- **Alternate preferred drug option:**
    - Nitazoxanide 500 mg PO BID x 3 days
- **Alternative antimicrobials:**
    - Paromomycin 500 mg PO TID x 5–10 days
    - Furazolidone 100 mg PO QID x 7–10 days
    - Quinacrine 100 mg PO TID x 5–7 days
    - Albendazole 400 mg PO Q-day x 5–7 days

Resistant strains of *Giardia* are increasingly prevalent, but many will retreat with a different class of antimicrobial therapy or a longer course of the original agent. In some refractory cases combination antimicrobial therapy may be necessary.

3. Cutaneous Leishmaniasis

Exposure Required:
- Bite from sand fly

Clinical Disease:
- Small papule that then forms a painless chronic ulcer with a raised indurated border

Diagnosis:
Organisms are found only in the living tissue at the raised margin, regardless of the age of the lesion.
- Histology
- Culture
- NAAT
- Leishmaniasis skin test

Treatment:
For non-mucocutaneous species (see mucocutaneous section for those species with mucocutaneous potential).

- **Physical Therapies**
    - Thermotherapy – 50 °C once weekly for 4 weeks
    - CO_2 laser – single session
    - Photodynamic therapy – once weekly for 4 weeks after application of 'photosensitizer'
    - Cryotherapy – freeze for 10–30 s, thaw and perform 2–3 times, repeated every 1–4 weeks for 2–4 sessions or more depending on response

- **Local Drug Therapy**
    - Paromomycin ointment 15% -apply BID for 20–28 days
    - Clotrimazole 1% / miconazole 2% ointment applied BID x 30 days
    - Intralesional antimonials (meglumine antimoniate injected until complete blanching of border, every 3–7 days for 1–5 sessions-very painful!)

- **Oral Drug Therapy**
    - Azoles
        - Fluconazole 400 mg PO Q-day x 6 weeks
        - Ketoconazole 600 mg PO Q-day x 6 weeks
        - Itraconazole 400 mg PO Q-day x 3–6 weeks
    - Miltefosine (2.5 mg/kg/day) or for an adult 150 mg PO per day given as 50 mg 2–3x/day x 28 days

- **Parenteral Therapy**
    - Pentavalent antimonials
    - Amphotericin
    - Liposomal amphotericin
    - Pentamidine

- **Combination Therapy**
    - Combining local and parenteral
    - Combining different parenteral therapies

4. Mucocutaneous Leishmaniasis

Leishmania (V.) braziliensis ~ 30%
Leishmania (V.) panamensis ~ 10%
Leishmania (V.) guyanensis ~ 10%
Leishmania (L.) amazonensis (rare)

Exposure Required:
- Bite from sand fly

Clinical Disease:
- Small papule that then forms a painless chronic ulcer with a raised indurated border, followed by ulcers at mucous membranes – i.e. soft palate, nasal septum, larynx, anus, lips

Diagnosis:
Organisms are found only in the living tissue at the raised margin, regardless of the age of the lesion.
- NAAT – main modality and identifies species
- Histology – very low sensitivity
- Culture – very low sensitivity

Treatment:
For species with muco-cutaneous potential, even first infection.
- **Oral Drug Therapy**
  - Miltefosine (2.5 mg/kg/day) or for an adult 150 mg PO per day given as 50 mg 2–3x/day x 28 days

- **Parenteral Therapy**
  - Pentavalent antimonials
    - Sodium stibogluconate 20 mg/kg/day IV/IM x 28–30 days
    - Meglumine antimoniate 20 mg/kg/day IV/IM x 28–30 days
  - Amphotericin 0.5–1 mg/kg IV Q-day up to cumulative dose of 20–45 mg/kg
  - Liposomal amphotericin 3 mg/kg IV Q-day up to cumulative dose of 20–60 mg/kg
  - (Possible inferior option) pentamidine 2–4 mg/kg IV/IM every other day or 3x/week for 15 doses

- **Combination Therapy**
  - Combining local and parenteral
  - Combining different parenteral therapies

5. Visceral Leishmaniasis
Leishmania (L.) donovani
Leishmania (L.) infantum

Exposure Required:
- Bite from sand fly

Clinical Disease:
- Fever, lymphadenopathy, hepatomegaly, splenomegaly, weight loss, darkening of the skin

Diagnosis:
- NAAT – from marrow or splenic aspirate
- Culture
- Microscopic evaluation
- rK39 antigen ELISA

Treatment:
- **Parenteral Therapy**
    - Liposomal amphotericin 3–5 mg/kg IV Q-day for 3–5 days up to cumulative dose of 15 mg/kg or single 10 mg/kg IV dose, for HIV co-infected 3–5 mg/kg IV Q-day for 10 days up to cumulative dose of 40 mg/kg
    - Pentavalent antimonials (preferred in Africa but not in India)
        - Sodium stibogluconate 20 mg/kg/day IV/IM x 28–30 days
        - Meglumine antimoniate 20 mg/kg/day IV/IM x 28–30 days
    - Amphotericin 0.5–1 mg/kg IV Q-day up to cumulative dose of 20–45 mg/kg
    - Liposomal amphotericin 3 mg/kg IV Q-day up to cumulative dose of 20–60 mg/kg

- **Oral Drug Therapy**
    - (Non-preferred-alternative) miltefosine (2.5 mg/kg/day) or for an adult 150 mg PO per day given as 50 mg 2–3x/day x 28 days

- **Combination Therapy**
    - Combining amphotericin and miltefosine

6. African Trypanosomiasis
Trypanosoma brucei rhodesiense
Trypanosoma brucei gambiense

Exposure Required:
- Bite from tsetse fly

Clinical Disease:
- Hemolymphatic stage – initially a large painless chancre at bite site, rash, generalized pruritus, weight loss, facial swelling, posterior cervical adenopathy
- CNS Stage – headache, stiff neck, periods of insomnia alternating with hypersomnolence, depression, seizures, tremors, palsies, coma

Diagnosis:
- Microscopic
    - Blood smears
    - Lymph node aspirates
    - CSF - examination of CSF is mandatory in the diagnostic evaluation of trypanosomiasis and a white blood cell count >5 cells/ml is considered indicative of CNS involvement
    - Aspirates taken at the edge of chancres
    - NAAT –limited availability
- Cultures
- Card agglutination test for trypanosomiasis

Treatment:
Treatment is determined by species and stage.
- **Early Stages:**
    Trypanosoma b. gambiense
    - (Preferred) pentamidine 4 mg/kg/day IV/IM (given over 2 hrs) for 7 days
    - (Alternative) suramin 100–200 mg test dose, then 20 mg/kg (max 1g) IV on days 1, 3, 7, 14, and 21

    Trypanosoma b. rhodesiense
    - Suramin 100–200 mg test dose, then 20 mg/kg (max 1g) IV on days 1, 3, 7, 14, and 21
- **Late Stages:**
    Trypanosoma b. gambiense
    - (Preferred) eflornithine 200 mg/kg IV q12 hrs (given over 1 hr) for 7 days PLUS nifurtimox 5 mg/kg PO q8 hrs for 10 days
    - Eflornithine 100 mg/kg IV q6 hrs for 14 days (monotherapy)
    - (Alternative) melarsoprol 2.2 mg/kg/day IV x 10 days (with oral prednisone)

    Trypanosoma b. rhodesiense
    - (Preferred) melarsoprol 2.2 mg/kg/day IV q10 days (with oral prednisone)
    - (Alternative) melarsoprol; three series of 3.6 mg/kg/day IV x 3 days spaced apart by 7-day intervals (with oral prednisone)

7. **American Trypanosomiasis**
    Trypanosoma cruzi

Exposure Required:
- Trypomastigotes present in reduviid bug feces enter through bug bite or mucous membranes, ingestion orally (contaminated sweetened drinks), transfusion, congenital

Clinical Disease:
- Acute – malaise, fever, myocarditis, pericardial effusion, meningoencephalitis
- Chronic – cardiac damage (arrhythmias, congestive heart failure), gastrointestinal (GI) damage (dysphagia, regurgitation, megacolon, constipation)

Diagnosis:
- Microscopic - blood smears
- NAAT - limited availability
- Serology
- Histology

Treatment:
- Benznidazole (for 60 days) through the Centers for Disease Control (CDC) and Prevention
    - Adults (>12 years old) 5–7.5 mg/kg daily divided into BID doses (12.5 and 100 mg tablets)
    - Children (< 12 years old) 5 mg/kg PO BID

- Nifurtimox (for 90 days) (divided into 3–4 doses per day)
    - Adults 8–10 mg/kg/day
    - Young children (<10 years old) 15–20 mg/kg/day
    - Older children (>10 years old <16 years old)12.5–15 mg/kg/day

8. *Trichomonas vaginalis*

Exposure Required:
- Acquisition of trophozoites during sexual contact or at birth

Clinical Disease:
- Asymptomatic
- Discomfort, dyspareunia, vaginal discharge (thick, yellow, blood tinged, pH increased from 4.5 to >5.0), strawberry cervix, erythema, dysuria

Diagnosis:
- Microscopic observation of motile forms from wet prep
- Culture
- Rapid antigen testing
- Nucleic acid probe test
- NAAT

Treatment:
- Metronidazole 500 mg PO BID x 7 days
- Tinidazole 2 g PO x1
- Combination: paromomycin compounded cream 250 mg each day with high dose tinidazole 1 g orally 3x/day for 2 weeks

9. The Malarias

Plasmodium falciparum
Plasmodium vivax
Plasmodium ovale
Plasmodium malariae
Plasmodium knowlesi

Exposure Required:
- Bite from female *Anopheles* mosquito

Clinical Disease:
- Periodic fever and chills, cough, abdominal pain, vomiting, diarrhea, dyspnea, anemia, leukopenia, eosinopenia, thrombocytopenia,

Diagnosis:
- Thick and thin blood smears
- Antibody-based rapid diagnostic tests
- NAAT
- Mutation-specific PCR

Staging:
- Uncomplicated malaria (not having a feature of severe)
- Severe malaria (having one or more of the following features)
    - Decreased level of consciousness
    - Unable to sit or stand without assistance
    - Convulsions (more than 2 in <24 hrs)
    - Acidosis or bicarbonate <15 mmol/L
    - Hypoglycemia (specific cutoffs)
    - Anemia (specific cutoffs)
    - Renal impairment (Cr >3 mg/dL or BUN >20 mmol/L
    - Jaundice (bilirubin >3 mg/dL)
    - Pulmonary edema (observable with chest X-ray, hypoxemia, tachypnea)
    - Significant bleeding
    - Shock
    - *P. falciparum* parasitemia >10%

Treatment:
- **Chloroquine-Sensitive Uncomplicated Malaria (not having a feature of severe)**
    - Chloroquine
        - Adults 1 g PO x1 then 500 mg at 6, 24, and 48 hrs
        - Children 10 mg/kg followed by 5 mg/kg of the base at 6, 24, and 48 hrs
    - Hydroxychloroquine
        - Adults 800 mg x1, then 400 mg at 6, 24, and 48 hrs
        - Children 10 mg/kg x1, then 5 mg/kg at 6, 24, and 48 hrs

- **Chloroquine-resistant Uncomplicated Malaria (not having a feature of severe)**
    - Artemisinin combination therapy (see table below)
    - Atovaquone-proguanil (adults) 4-tablets PO Q-Day x 3 days
    - Quinine 650 mg PO TID for 3–7 days plus second agent for 7 days PLUS (doxycycline, or tetracycline, or clindamycin)
    - Mefloquine 3-tablets PO x1, then 2 tablets 6 hrs later

- **Treatment of Complicated Malaria**
    - Artemisinin derivatives
        - Artesunate IV (preferred) (If >20 kg) 2.4 mg/kg IV x1 then at 12 hrs, 24 hrs, then daily, (If <20 kg) 3 mg/kg IV same schedule
        - Artemether IM 3.2 mg/kg IM x1 then 1.6 mg/kg Q-day
    - Quinidine based
        - Quinidine gluconate 10 mg/kg IV x1 then continuous infusion 0.0125 mg/kg/min
        - Plus, doxycycline or clindamycin for 7 days

- **Treatment to Prevent Malaria Relapse (Hyponozoites)**
    - Primaquine – 30 mg (of base) 2-tablets PO Q-day for 2 weeks

Consider broad spectrum antibiotics (~10% coinfected)/Exchange transfusion not recommended

Medication	Forms available	Weight (kg)-Dose(mg)
Artemether-lumefantrine	20/120mg 40/240mg	<15kg 20/120, 15-25kg 40/240, 25-35kg 60/360, >35kg 80/480 (PO BID x 3 days)
Artesunate-amodiaquine	25/67.5mg 50/135mg 100/270mg and separate tablets	<9kg 25/67.5, 9-18kg 50/135, 18-36kg 100/270, >36kg 200/540 (PO Q-day x 3 days)
Artesunate-mefloquine	25/55mg 100/220mg and separate tablets	<9kg 25/55, 9-18kg 50/110, 18-30kg 100/220, >30kg 200/440 (PO Q-day x 3 days)
Artesunate-sulfadoxine-pyrimethamine	Artesunate(A) 50mg and SP 500/25mg	<10kg SP-250/12.5 PO x1 day#1+A-25 PO Q-day x 3days, 10-25kg SP-500/25 PO x1 day#1+A-50 PO Q-day x 3days, 25-50kg SP-1000/50 PO x1 day#1+A-100 PO Q-day x 3days, >50kg SP-1500/75 PO x1 day#1+A-200 PO Q-day x 3days
Dihydroartemisinin-piperaquine	20/160mg 40/320mg and separate tablets	<8kg 20/160, 8-11kg 30/240, 11-17kg 40/320 17-25kg 60/480, 25-36kg 80/640, 36-60 120/960, 60-80kg 160/1280, >80kg 200/1600 (PO Q-day x 3days)

10. *Cryptosporidium parvum*

Exposure Required:
- Oral ingestion of oocysts in fecally contaminated water or food, rarely aerosol

Clinical Disease:
- Watery diarrhea, upper abdominal cramps, anorexia, nausea, weight loss and vomiting

Diagnosis:
- Stool microscopy
- PCR testing
- Antigen tests
- Multiplex NAAT testing

Treatment:
Limited evidence for benefit from any specific therapy so main focus is on restoration of immune dysfunction, if present, and rehydration.

- Nitazoxanide 500 mg PO TID for 3–14 days

11. *Toxoplasma gondii*

Exposure Required:
- Oral ingestion of pseudocysts in undercooked or raw meat, or oocysts from cat feces, and vertical transmission from mother to child during pregnancy

Clinical Disease:
- Congenital – chorioretinitis, hydrocephalus, intracranial calcifications, hepatomegaly, liver failure, thrombocytopenia, seizures, cognitive deficiencies
- Acute – mono-like illness, fever, cervical adenopathy, fatigue
- Reactivation in immunocompromised patient – encephalitis, ring enhancing cerebral lesions, interstitial pneumonitis

Diagnosis:
- Microscopy
- NAAT
- Specific immunoglobulins
- Imaging

Treatment:
- (If < 60kg) pyrimethamine 100–200 mg x1 then 50 mg PO daily + sulfadiazine 1,000 mg PO QID + leukovorin 10–25 mg PO daily
- (If > 60 kg) pyrimethamine 100–200 mg x1 then 75 mg PO daily + sulfadiazine 1,500 mg PO QID + leukovorin 10–25 mg PO daily
- (If pyrimethamine is unavailable then TMP-SMX 5 mg/kg based on TMP component IV/PO BID)
- Pregnancy- unclear on best approach but spiramycin has been used during the first trimester

12. *Entamoeba histolytica*

Exposure Required:
- Oral ingestion of cysts in fecally contaminated water or food

Clinical Disease:
- Intestinal – acute bloody diarrhea (dysentery but blood may only be microscopic), less commonly chronic diarrhea, abdominal discomfort, amoeboma (colonic mass)
- Extra-intestinal – liver lesions, pulmonary lesion, less commonly (pleura, cardiac and cerebral)

Diagnosis:
- Antigens
- NAAT
- Microscopy coupled with species identification by one of the first two testing modalities

Treatment:
- **Intestinal**
    - (Preferred) metronidazole 500 mg PO TID for 10 days
    - (Alternative) tinidazole 2 g PO Q-day x 3 days
    - (Alternative) nitazoxanide 500 mg PO BID x 3 days
    - (Luminal agents) iodoquinol 650 mg PO TID x 20 days or, paromomycin 1,000 mg PO TID x 7 days or diloxanide 500 mg PO TID x 10 days
- **Extra-intestinal**
    - (Preferred) metronidazole 500 mg PO TID for 10 days
    - (Alternative) tinidazole 2 g PO Q-day x 5 days
    - (Alternative) nitazoxanide 500 mg PO BID x 10 days
    - (Luminal agents) iodoquinol 650 mg PO TID x 20 days or, paromomycin 1,000 mg PO TID x 7 days or diloxanide 500 mg PO TID x 10 days

13. *Balantidium coli*

Exposure Required:
- Oral ingestion of cysts in fecally contaminated water or food

Clinical Disease:
- Asymptomatic, watery diarrhea, dysentery, fever, nausea, vomiting, malaise

Diagnosis:
- Microscopy

Treatment:
- Tetracycline 500 mg PO 4x/day x 10 days
- Metronidazole 750 mg PO TID x 5 days
- Iodoquinol, paromomycin, nitazoxanide and chloroquine have been used

14. Other Protozoa of Medical Importance

A. *Babesia spp.*

Exposure Required:
- Bite of larval *Ixodes scapularis* tick (black legged deer tick)

Clinical Disease:
- Fever, malaise, headache, bradycardia, lymphopenia, anemia

Diagnosis:
- Microscopy (blood smears) rarely a 'Maltese cross' can be seen
- NAAT
- Serology

Treatment:
- **Immunocompetent**
    - Mild to Moderate Disease:
        - (Preferred) azithromycin 500 mg PO day 1 then 250 mg PO Q-day PLUS atovaquone 750 mg PO BID for 7–10 days
        - (Alternative) clindamycin 600 mg PO TID PLUS quinine 650 mg PO TID for 7–10 days
    - Severe Disease (consider exchange transfusion):
        - (Preferred) azithromycin 500 mg IV Q-day PLUS atovaquone 750 mg PO BID for 7–10 days
        - (Alternative) clindamycin 300–600 mg IV TID PLUS quinine 650 mg PO TID for 7–10 days

- **Immunocompromised**
    - Mild to Moderate Disease:
        - (Preferred) azithromycin 1000 mg PO Q-day PLUS atovaquone 750 mg PO BID for 7–10 days or longer
        - (Alternative) clindamycin 600 mg PO TID PLUS quinine 650 mg PO TID for 7–10 days or longer

- o Severe Disease (consider exchange transfusion):
    - (Preferred) azithromycin 500 mg IV Q-day PLUS atovaquone 750 mg PO BID for 7–10 days or longer
    - (Alternative) clindamycin 300–600 mg IV TID PLUS quinine 650 mg PO TID for 7–10 days or longer

B. *Cystoisospora belli*

Exposure Required:
- Oral ingestion of oocysts in fecally contaminated water or food (not direct person to person as 1–2 days required for sporulation)

Clinical Disease:
- Fever, abdominal cramping, watery non-bloody diarrhea, malaise, weight loss, eosinophilia

Diagnosis:
- Stool microscopy –requires acid fast staining or specific fluorescent techniques
- NAAT

Treatment:
- **Immunocompetent**
    - o Trimethoprim-sulfamethoxazole (TMP-SMX) double strength 160/800 mg PO BID for 7–10 days
- **Immunocompromised**
    - o (Preferred) trimethoprim-sulfamethoxazole (TMP-SMX) double strength 160/800 mg PO BID for 14 days followed by 1-tab PO 3 times per week
    - o (Alternative-inferior) pyrimethamine with leucovorin or nitazoxanide may have activity
    - o (Alternative-inferior) ciprofloxacin 500 mg PO BID for 14 days

C. *Cyclospora cayetanensis*

Exposure Required:
- Oral ingestion of oocysts in fecally contaminated water or food

Clinical Disease:
- Watery diarrhea

Diagnosis:
- Microscopy (improved sensitivity with acid-fast staining)
- NAAT

Treatment:
- (Preferred) trimethoprim-sulfamethoxazole (TMP-SMX) double strength 160/800 mg PO BID for 7–10 days
- (Alternative) nitazoxanide 500 mg PO BID for 7 days
- (Alternative-inferior) ciprofloxacin 500 mg PO BID x 7 days

D. *Naeglaria fowleri*

Exposure Required:
- Contact of the inside of the nasal cavity (cribriform plate) with water containing trophozoites

Clinical Disease:
- Frontal headache, vomiting, confusion, fever, coma

Diagnosis:
- Microscopy/histology
- NAAT

Treatment: (multidrug regimen)
- Conventional-amphotericin (not liposomal) 1.5 mg/kg/day IV, and
- Rifampin 10 mg/kg/day PO in three doses, and
- Fluconazole 10 mg/kg/day IV or PO, and
- Miltefosine 50 mg PO BID or TID, and
- Azithromycin 500 mg Q-day IV or PO

E. *Acanthamoeba* spp.

Exposure Required:
- Most likely acquired through lungs or skin on exposure to keratitis contaminated tap water

Clinical Disease:
- Encephalitic form- Granulomatous Amebic Encephalitis (GAE) - frontal headache, diplopia, seizures
- Ulcerative keratitis – gritty feeling in eye, impaired vision, blindness

Diagnosis:
- Microscopy identification of trophozoites on wet mount, by confocal, or in fixed specimens
- Culture
- NAAT

Treatment:
- Keratitis – often combination therapy
- Disseminated disease (skin, CNS, disseminated) – use combination therapy

F. *Balamuthia mandrillaris*

Exposure Required:
- Acquired through lungs or skin

Clinical Disease:
- Fever, stiff neck, headache, encephalitis

Diagnosis:
- Microscopy/histology (immunofluorescent antibodies available)
- NAAT

Treatment:
- Multi-drug regimens containing 4–5 agents such as amphotericin, fluconazole, albendazole and miltefosine
- (Additional alternative agents) voriconazole, flucytosine, pentamidine, azithromycin, clarithromycin, trimethoprim-sulfamethoxazole and sulfadiazine

G. *Blastocystis hominis*

Exposure Required:
- Oral ingestion of cysts in fecally contaminated water or food

Clinical Disease:
- Asymptomatic, diarrhea, abdominal discomfort

Diagnosis:
- Stool microscopy
- NAAT

Treatment:
- Metronidazole 500 mg PO TID for 5–10 days
- Tinidazole 2 g PO x1
- Paromomycin 500 mg PO TID for 7–10 days
- Trimethoprim-sulfamethoxazole (TMP-SMX) double strength 160/800 mg PO BID for 7 days
- Nitazoxanide 500 mg PO BID for 3 days

H. *Dientamoeba fragilis*

Exposure Required:
- Oral ingestion of fecally contaminated water or food

Clinical Disease:
- Diarrhea, nausea, abdominal discomfort

Diagnosis:
- Stool microscopy –issues with sensitivity
- NAAT

Treatment:
- Metronidazole 500 mg PO TID for 10 days
- Paromomycin 10 mg/kg PO TID for 7 days
- Iodoquinol 650 mg PO TID for 20 days
- Tetracycline 400 mg PO QID for 10 days
- Doxycycline 100 mg PO BID for 10 days

15. Non-pathogenic Protozoa

- Commensal flagellates – no treatment
- Commensal amoebae – no treatment

16. *Enterobius vermicularis*

Exposure Required:
- Oral ingestion of embryonated eggs, autoinfection

Clinical Disease:
- Asymptomatic, perianal pruritus, vaginal irritation

Diagnosis:
- Microscopy - pinworm paddle or clear adhesive tape to collect eggs, not standard O+P, and direct visualization of adult females
- NAAT

Treatment:
Treatment of exposed contacts, all household members, and/or source patients, if not household members, is recommended and has been successful in both households and institutions.

- Pyrantel pamoate 11 mg/kg PO x1 then repeated 2–3 weeks later
- Albendazole 400 mg PO x1 then repeated 2–3 weeks later
- Mebendazole 100 mg PO x1 then repeated 2–3 weeks later
- (Inferior option) ivermectin 200 mcg/kg PO x 1 then repeated 2–3 weeks later

17. *Trichuris trichiura*

Exposure Required:
- Oral ingestion of embryonated eggs

Clinical Disease:
- Asymptomatic, dysentery, tenesmus, weight loss, anemia, rectal prolapse

Diagnosis:
- Stool microscopy - standard O+P and direct visualization of adults on endoscopy
- NAAT

Treatment:
- (Preferred) mebendazole 100 mg PO BID x 3 days
- (Inferior option) albendazole 400 mg PO Q-day x 3 days
- (Inferior option) ivermectin 200 mcg/kg PO x 1

18. *Ascaris lumbricoides*

Exposure Required:
- Oral ingestion of embryonated eggs

Clinical Disease:
- Migratory phase – Löeffler's syndrome -pneumonitis, hepatomegaly, bronchospasm, eosinophilia
- Intestinal phase – asymptomatic, high burden can lead to obstruction, aberrant migration can lead to peritonitis or obstruction such as in hepatobiliary ascariasis

Diagnosis:
- Stool microscopy - standard O+P and direct visualization of adults on endoscopy
- NAAT

Treatment:
- Albendazole 400 mg PO x 1
- Mebendazole 500 mg PO x 1 or 100 mg PO BID for 3 days
- Pyrantel pamoate 11 mg/kg PO x1 (can be used during pregnancy)
- (Inferior option) ivermectin 200 mcg/kg PO x 1

19. **The Hookworms**
Necator americanus
Ancylostoma duodenale
Ancylostoma ceylanicum

Exposure Required:
- Infective L3 filariform larvae penetrate skin (usually through a hair follicle) *Ancyclostoma duodenale* larvae are also infective orally

Clinical Disease:
- Dermatitis-(during entry), pneumonia-(during migratory phase), abdominal pain-(can occur with heavy oral ingestion with eosinophilia 'Wakana disease'), chronic iron deficiency anemia, skin pigmentation change to yellow-green 'chlorosis'-(chronic disease)

Diagnosis:
- Stool microscopy - standard O+P and direct visualization of adults on endoscopy
- NAAT

Treatment:
Ivermectin has poor efficacy and is not recommended.
- (Preferred) albendazole 400 mg PO x 1
- Mebendazole 500 mg PO x 1 or 100 mg PO BID x 1 day
- Pyrantel pamoate 11 mg/kg PO Q-day x 3 days

20. *Strongyloides stercoralis*

Exposure Required:
- Infective L3 filariform larvae penetrate skin (usually through a hair follicle)

Clinical Disease:
- Asymptomatic, watery diarrhea, eosinophilia, dermatitis-('ground itch'), *larva currens* rash, periumbilical thumbprint purpura rash, with hyperinfection-bacterial sepsis and bacterial meningitis, with *S. fuelleborni* swollen belly syndrome

Diagnosis:
- Microscopy - stool O+P but larvae are seen not eggs, or histological examination of tissues
- Fecal culture - coproculture
- Serology
- NAAT

Treatment:
Control (not elimination)
- **Uncomplicated Infection:**
    - Ivermectin 200 mcg/kg/day given once and then repeated 2 weeks later (so for 60 kg adult 4 of the 3 mg tablets PO each time)
    - (Inferior alternative) albendazole 400 mg PO Q-day for 7-days
- **Disseminated Disease:**
    - Ivermectin 200 mcg/kg/day PO Q-day with duration determined by clinical response, some will add albendazole 400 mg PO Q-day if poor clinical response (Some patients have been successfully treated off label with subcutaneous dosing of veterinarian ivermectin preparations).

21. *Trichinella spiralis*

Exposure Required:
- Oral ingestion of raw or undercooked meats

Clinical Disease:
- Gastrointestinal phase – secretory diarrhea, abdominal pain, nausea, vomiting
- Parenteral phase – fever, myalgia, bilateral periorbital edema, petechial hemorrhages, leukocytosis, eosinophilia, can have CNS or cardiac involvement with meningoencephalitis or arrythmias

Diagnosis:
- Microscopy - histological examination of tissues after muscle biopsy
- Serology - ELISA with Western blot confirmation
- NAAT
- Supportive laboratory tests – muscle enzymes, such as creatine kinase, lactic dehydrogenase, and peripheral eosinophilia

Treatment:
- Albendazole 400 mg PO BID x 14 days
- Mebendazole 400 mg PO TID x 14 days
- Prednisone 30–60 mg Q-day for 14 days (add to regimen only if diagnosis secure)
- Antipyretics and analgesics

22. Lymphatic Filariae
Wuchereria bancrofti
Brugia malayi

Exposure Required:
- Bite from mosquito (wide variety of genera and species)

Clinical Disease:
- Asymptomatic – lymphatic dilation detectable only by ultrasound or other testing
- Acute lymphadenitis – fever, painful swelling of lymph nodes, secondary bacterial infections
- Elephantiasis – lymphedema of arms, legs, breasts, genitalia, secondary bacterial infections
- Tropical pulmonary eosinophilia – nocturnal asthma with dyspnea, fatigue, weight loss, and eosinophilia

Diagnosis:
- Microscopy - of blood smears during the night and can be concentrated
- Serology - ELISA with Western blot confirmation
- Antigen testing – circulating filarial antigen assay
- NAAT - research tool, no commercially available tests
- Ultrasound – lymphatic vessels and can detect filarial dance sign in the spermatic cord

Treatment:
It is critical that, prior to treatment, co-infection with *Loa loa* with a high *Loa loa* microfilarial load is ruled out, due to the risk of severe adverse events if treatment is given to such patients.
- **Antiparasitics:**
    - Diethylcarbamazine (DEC) 6 mg/kg/day x 12 days for a total of 72 mg/kg body weight
    - Doxycycline 100 mg PO BID for 6 weeks
    - Ivermectin as part of mass drug programs
    - Albendazole as part of mass drug programs
- **Surgery:** hydrocele drainage and lymphatic surgery
- **Complementary care:**
    - Lymphedema care
    - Treatment of wounds and secondary bacterial infections

23. *Onchocerca volvulus*

Exposure Required:
- Bite of the black fly (*Simulium* spp.)

Clinical Disease:
- Dermatitis – papular changes (can be extremely pruritic), lichenification (*sowda*), atrophy (hanging groin), depigmentation (leopard skin), reddish facial lesions (*erysipelas de la costa*)
- Lymphadenopathy – Africa (inguinal), Americas (head and neck)
- Ocular – keratitis, iritis, optic atrophy, optic neuritis, cataracts, chorioretinitis, blindness
- Nodding syndrome – not clearly caused by this parasite but presents with seizures, head nodding, periods of unresponsiveness, long-term disability

Diagnosis:
- Microscopy - bloodless skin snips, blood smears to rule out other infections
- Serology - ELISA with Western blot confirmation
- Mazzotti test - now modified test
- NAAT - research tool, no commercially available tests
- Ultrasound - evaluation of nodules

Treatment:
The major toxicity of ivermectin is generally not from the drug itself but rather from its ability to increase the antigen load from dead and dying parasites, leading to fever, angioedema and pruritus. These symptoms usually occur within 24 hrs of treatment. In those patients with concurrent *Loa loa* infection, ivermectin can elicit severe reactions, including encephalopathy and consequently it is essential to evaluate the patients in areas endemic for *Loa loa* for co-infection.
- **Endemic Area:**
    - Ivermectin 150 mcg/kg by mouth every 6 months for years
    - (Alternative) doxycycline 100 mg PO 1x/day x 6 weeks followed by ivermectin
- **Outside Endemic Area:**
    - Ivermectin 150 mcg/kg by mouth every 6 months for several years until asymptomatic
    - (Alternative) doxycycline 100 mg PO 1x/day x 6 weeks followed by ivermectin

24. *Loa loa*

Exposure Required:
- Bite from the deer fly (*Chrysops* spp.)

Clinical Disease:
- Asymptomatic, Calabar swellings, angioedema, localized swelling, worm migration across eye, cardiomyopathy, renal disease, encephalitis, lymphadenitis, eosinophilia, -serious adverse reactions when treated for other parasitic infections

Diagnosis:
- Microscopy - of blood smears during the middle of the day and can be concentrated
- Serology - ELISA with Western blot confirmation
- NAAT - research tool, no commercially available tests

Treatment:

It is critical that, prior to treatment, co-infection with *L. loa* with a high *L. loa* microfilarial load is ruled out, due to the risk of severe adverse events if treatment is given to such patients.
- **>2,500 microfilariae/ml**: If levels are greater than 2,500 mf/ml, then apheresis or treatment with albendazole 200 mg PO BID until loads <2,500 mf/ml.
- **<2,500 microfilariae/ml**:
    - Diethylcarbamazine (DEC)
        - CDC regimen: DEC 8 to 10 mg/kg/day in 3 divided doses for 21 days; patients with symptomatic loiasis and microfilarial loads ≥ 8,000 mf/mL should receive apheresis or treatment with albendazole prior to treatment with diethylcarbamazine (CDC 2015). For patients with microfilaria in the blood, some clinicians recommend the following dose-escalating regimen: 50 mg as a single dose on day 1; 50 mg 3 times daily on day 2; 100 mg 3 times daily on day 3; 9 mg/kg/day in 3 divided doses on day 4 to end of treatment course. Repeat courses of treatment may be needed to achieve cure.
        - World Health Organization recommendations: DEC 1 mg/kg as a single dose on day 1, with doubling of the dose on the next 2 days, then 6–9 mg/kg/day in divided doses 3 times daily for 18 days.
- **Surgery:** Adult worms in the eye can be removed surgically.
- **Albendazole:** Alternatives to DEC include albendazole 200 mg PO BID x 21 days that can effectively reduce the number of circulating microfilariae by acting directing on adult worms.
- Ivermectin is not a preferred agent for the treatment of loiasis and can be associated with significant morbidity if given to patients with high levels of circulating microfilariae.
- Chemoprophylaxis with weekly DEC given in a dose of 300 mg is effective in preventing loiasis among long-term visitors but is not currently recommended for short-term visitors to endemic areas.

25. *Dracunculus medinensis*

Exposure Required:
- Oral ingestion of infected copepods

Clinical Disease:
- Cutaneous blisters and ulcers, allergic reactions and superinfection with failed attempts to remove worms, arthritis, contractures and scarring causing disability and absenteeism from work and school

Diagnosis:
- Direct visualization: locating head of the adult worm in the skin lesion
- Microscopy - identifying the larvae that are released into freshwater
- ELISA - availability limited
- Radiographs - calcifications corresponding to adult worms

Treatment:
- Slow mechanical extraction of about 1cm/day, pain control and treatment of any secondary bacterial infections

26. Other Nematodes of Medical Importance

A. *Capillaria hepatica*

Exposure Required:
- Oral ingestion of embryonated eggs

Clinical Disease:
- Asymptomatic, liver failure, abdominal lymphadenopathy, eosinophilia

Diagnosis:
- Histology - after liver biopsy or at autopsy
- Serological testing - ELISA and indirect fluorescent antibody test (IFA), high sensitivity and specificity but not widely available

Treatment:
- Combination therapy has been used successfully with combinations of albendazole, thiabendazole, disophenol (2-6-diiodo-4-nitrophenol) and prednisone

B. *Capillaria philippinensis*

Exposure Required:
- Oral ingestion of raw or undercooked freshwater fish or crustaceans

Clinical Disease:
- Diarrhea

Diagnosis:
- Stool microscopy - standard O+P with direct visualization of eggs or larvae in stool or detecting the adults on small bowel biopsy of the small intestinal wall

Treatment:
- Albendazole 400 mg PO Q-day x 30 days
- Mebendazole 200 mg PO BID x 20–30 days

C. *Dirofilaria immitis*

Exposure Required:
- Bite of infected mosquito

Clinical Disease:
- Coin lesion in lung

Diagnosis:
- Histology
- Radiographs - coin lesion in lungs

Treatment:
No known effective therapies in humans

D. *Mansonella ozzardi*

Exposure Required:
- Bite of black flies and biting midges

Clinical Disease:
- Asymptomatic, urticaria, lymphadenopathy, chronic arthritis, eosinophilia

Diagnosis:
- Microscopy - visualization of microfilariae in a blood smear, sensitivity increased with concentration techniques
- ELISA - based on crude antigen preparations but with limited specificity
- PCR - developed and available through the National Institutes of Health

Treatment:
- Ivermectin 200 mcg/kg/day PO x1

E. *Mansonella perstans*

Exposure Required:
- Bite from biting midge

Clinical Disease:
- Asymptomatic, painless conjunctival nodules, eyelid swelling, angioedema, (called the Ugandan or Kampala eye worm)

Diagnosis:
- Microscopy - visualization of microfilariae in a blood smear, sensitivity increased with concentration techniques
- ELISA - based on crude antigen preparations but with limited specificity
- PCR - developed and available through the National Institutes of Health

Treatment:
Considered one of the most challenging filarial infections to treat.
- Combination therapy has been successful
- Doxycycline has been successfully used on strains from Mozambique and the Democratic Republic of Congo that harbor the endosymbiont Wolbachia

F. *Mansonella streptocerca*

Exposure Required:
- Biting midges

Clinical Disease:
- Pruritic dermatitis, hypopigmented macules

Diagnosis:
- Microscopy - visualization of microfilariae in a blood smear, sensitivity increased with concentration techniques
- ELISA - based on crude antigen preparations but with limited specificity
- PCR - developed and available through the National Institutes of Health

Treatment:
- Diethylcarbamazine (DEC) 2 mg/kg/day TID for 12 days
- Ivermectin 150 mcg/kg/day PO x1 can reduce microfilarial levels

G. *Oesophagostomum bifurcum*

Exposure Required:
- Oral ingestion of infective larvae

Clinical Disease:
- Asymptomatic, abdominal nodules or masses, abdominal pain

Diagnosis:
- Stool microscopy - standard O+P with direct visualization of eggs (cannot be visually distinguished from hookworm eggs)
- Coproculture - allowing eggs to develop to third stage larvae (difficult and time consuming)
- Histology of biopsied nodules showing larval or adult forms
- Imaging - Ultrasound
- NAAT - PCR/Multiplex

Treatment:
- Pyrantel pamoate 11mg/kg PO x1
- Albendazole 400 mg PO x1

H. *Ternidens diminutus*

Exposure Required:
- Oral ingestion of infective larvae

Clinical Disease:
- Colonic ulcerations, nodular lesions, abdominal mass

Diagnosis:
- Stool microscopy - standard O+P with direct visualization of eggs (can not be visually distinguished from hookworm eggs)

Treatment:
- Pyrantel pamoate 11 mg/kg PO x1
- Albendazole 400 mg PO x1

27. Aberrant Nematode Infections

A. Cutaneous Larva Migrans

Exposure Required:
- Infective larvae penetrate unbroken skin

Clinical Disease:
- Serpiginous lesions, pruritus, secondary bacterial infections

Diagnosis:
- Physical findings: visualization of serpiginous lesions
- Dermoscopy - translucent brown areas and red-dotted vessels

Treatment:
- (Preferred) Ivermectin 200 mcg/kg PO Q-day x 1–2 days
- (Alternative) Albendazole 400 mg PO Q-day x 3–7 days
- Topical thiabendazole 15% applied daily for 5 days
- Topical albendazole ointment 10% applied TID x 10 days

B. Visceral Larva Migrans

Exposure Required:
- Oral ingestion of embryonated eggs

Clinical Disease:
- Tissue damage, cognitive defects, hypersensitivity responses, eosinophilia

Diagnosis:
- Serology - ELISA
- NAAT - research tool, no commercially available tests
- Ophthalmological exam for ocular larva migrans (OLM)
- Imaging - CT, MRI, Ultrasound

Treatment:
- Steroids for severe or CNS reactions
- Albendazole 400 mg PO BID x 5 days

C. Ocular Larva Migrans

Exposure Required:
- Oral ingestion of embryonated eggs

Clinical Disease:
- Ocular granulomas, visual disturbance, blindness

Diagnosis:
- Serology - ELISA

Treatment:
- Steroids for some ophthalmic or CNS reactions
- Albendazole 400 mg PO BID x 5 days
- Surgery (vitrectomy)

D. *Baylisascaris procyonis*

Exposure Required:
- Oral ingestion of embryonated eggs

Clinical Disease:
- Nausea, fatigue, hepatomegaly, loss of coordination and muscle control, eosinophilic meningitis, ocular disease, encephalitis, coma

Diagnosis:
- Serology - recombinant protein-based ELISA

Treatment:
- Albendazole 25–50 mg/kg/day in divided doses x 20 days, with concomitant steroids

E. *Angiostrongylus cantonensis/costaricensis*

Exposure Required:
- Oral ingestion of infective larvae

Clinical Disease:
- *A. cantonensis* - eosinophilic meningoencephalitis, fever, headache, painful paresthesias
- *A. costaricensis* – abdominal pain, fever, nausea, vomiting

Diagnosis:
- CSF examination for eosinophilia
- PCR of CSF fluid
- Imaging - MRI may reveal areas of enhancement in characteristic patterns
- Serology - ELISA (not widely available and older assays cross react with gnathostomiasis)

Treatment:
- Analgesics, repeated lumbar punctures, steroids and albendazole are used but optimal treatment is not defined

F. *Gnathostoma spinigerum*

Exposure Required:
- Ingestion of infective larvae in fish, snakes, and birds

Clinical Disease:
- Asymptomatic, cutaneous larva migrans, subcutaneous swellings, eosinophilic meningitis, painful paresthesias

Diagnosis:
- CSF examination for eosinophilia
- Imaging - MRI may reveal areas of enhancement in characteristic patterns and CT may demonstrate areas of hemorrhage
- Serology - ELISA (not widely available and older assays cross react with *Angiostrongylus cantonensis*)

Treatment:
- Albendazole 400 mg PO Q-day x 21 days
- Ivermectin 200 mcg/kg PO Q-day x 2 days
- Repeated lumbar punctures to reduce opening pressure, steroids

G. *Anisakiasis*

Exposure Required:
- Oral ingestion of infective larvae in raw or undercooked saltwater fish or squid

Clinical Disease:
- Abdominal pain, nausea, vomiting, diarrhea, fever

Diagnosis:
- Direct visualization of parasites by endoscopy or in vomit
- Serology - ELISA
- PCR - not commercially available outside research settings

Treatment:
- Physical removal of the parasite prior to penetration
- Surgery after penetration
- Albendazole 400 mg PO BID for 3–21 days but optimal therapy is not defined

28. *Taenia saginata*

Exposure Required:
- Ingestion of raw or undercooked beef containing cysticerci

Clinical Disease:
- Asymptomatic, proglottids noted in stool or clothing

Diagnosis:
- Microscopy:
  - Gravid proglottids can be fixed in 10% formaldehyde solution, and the uterus injected with India ink, with the aid of a 26-gauge needle or stained with hematoxylin-eosin staining techniques. *T. saginata* proglottids have 12 or more branches on either side of the uterus.
  - Eggs of *T. saginata* are occasionally found in stool, since most proglottids usually pass out of the host intact. If an egg is seen on stool examination, the species cannot be determined on visual microscopy based on morphology, since all members of the family Taeniidae produce visually identical ova. Upon acid-fast staining, occasionally the species can be distinguished, as fully mature eggs of *T. saginata* have an acid-fast shell.
  - Paddle Test/Sticky Tape Test is an additional diagnostically relevant test (see: diagnosis for *Enterobius vermicularis*). When proglottids migrate out of the anus, they express eggs that remain on the perineum.
- NAAT – PCR/ loop-mediated isothermal amplification (LAMP)/Multiplex
- Antigen detection (coproantigens) – used on stool samples

Treatment:
- Praziquantel 5–10 mg/kg PO x1 (600 mg tablets)
- Niclosamide 2 g PO x1 (not commercially available in the United States)

29. *Taenia solium*

Intestinal

Exposure Required:
- Ingestion of raw or undercooked pork containing cysticerci

Clinical Disease:
- Asymptomatic, proglottids noted in stool or clothing

Diagnosis:
- Microscopy:
  - Gravid proglottids can be fixed in 10% formaldehyde solution, and the uterus injected with India ink, with the aid of a 26-gauge needle or stained with hematoxylin-eosin staining techniques. *T. solium* proglottids have less than 12 branches on either side of the uterus.

- o Eggs of *T. solium* are occasionally found in stool, since most proglottids usually pass out of the host intact. If an egg is seen on stool examination, the species cannot be determined on visual microscopy based on morphology, since all members of the family Taeniidae produce visually identical ova. Upon acid-fast staining, occasionally the species can be distinguished, as fully mature eggs of *T. saginata* have an acid-fast shell and *T. solium* eggs have a shell that is not acid-fast.
- o Paddle Test/Sticky Tape Test is an additional diagnostically relevant test (see: diagnosis for *Enterobius vermicularis*). When proglottids migrate out of the anus, they express eggs that remain on the perineum.
- NAAT - PCR/ loop-mediated isothermal amplification (LAMP)/Multiplex
- Antigen detection (coproantigens) - used on stool samples

Treatment:
- Praziquantel 5–10 mg/kg PO x1 (600 mg tablets)
- Niclosamide 2 g PO x1 (not commercially available in the United States)

Extra-intestinal (Cysticercosis and Neurocysticercosis)

Exposure Required:
- Oral ingestion of embryonated eggs

Clinical Disease:
- Extraneural – subcutaneous (discrete swellings that go on to become tender), intramuscular (asymptomatic, cysts in muscles, calcifications)
- Neurocysticercosis – intraparenchymal/extraparenchymal (space occupying symptoms, headaches, seizures, hydrocephalus, focal neurological abnormalities)

Diagnosis:
- Imaging - recommend that patients undergo both MRI and CT for CNS disease, plain radiographs can also show peripheral calcified disease
- Serology - Enzyme-linked immune-transfer blot, rather than crude antigen assays
- NAAT - PCR/ loop mediated isothermal amplification (LAMP) /Multiplex

Treatment:
- Monotherapy for 1–2 viable cysts - albendazole 7.5 mg/kg PO BID for 10 days (200 mg tablets)
- Combination therapy for > 2 viable cysts - albendazole 7.5 mg/kg PO BID for 10 days (200 mg tablets) and praziquantel 5 mg/kg PO TID for 10 days (600 mg tablets)
- Corticosteroids (recommended for all CNS disease when using antiparasitics) - prednisone 1 mg/kg PO Q-day x 5–10 days then tapered or dexamethasone 10 mg IV x1 then 4 mg IV q6 hrs x 5–10 days then tapered. For acute encephalitis steroids alone without antiparasitics are recommended.
- Antiepileptic therapy - recommended for all patients having seizures
- Mechanical therapy - for extraparenchymal neurocysticercosis surgical therapy and ventriculoperitoneal shunting may be required.

30. *Diphyllobothrium latum*

Exposure Required:
- Oral ingestion of infective larvae from eating raw or undercooked freshwater or andromous fish

Clinical Disease:
- Asymptomatic, watery diarrhea, fatigue, B12 deficiency

Diagnosis:
- Microscopy:
    - Gravid proglottids can be fixed in 10% formaldehyde solution, and stained with hematoxylin-eosin staining techniques. These proglottids are wider than they are long (most proglottids do not pass out of the host intact).
    - Eggs can be found in stool (most proglottids do not pass out of the host intact)
- NAAT

Treatment:
- Praziquantel 5–10 mg/kg PO x1 (600 mg tablets)
- Niclosamide 2 g PO x1 (not commercially available in the United States)

31. Other Tapeworms of Medical Importance

A. *Hymenolepis nana*

Exposure Required:
- Oral ingestion of infective larvae along with infected insect or oral ingestion of embryonated eggs

Clinical Disease:
- Asymptomatic, rarely diarrhea

Diagnosis:
- Standard detection of eggs on stool O+P

Treatment:
- Praziquantel 5–10 mg/kg PO x1 (600 mg tablets)
- (Inferior alternative) nitazoxanide 500 mg PO BID x 3 days

B. *Hymenolepis diminuta*

Exposure Required:
- Oral ingestion of infective larvae along with infected insect

Clinical Disease:
- Asymptomatic

Diagnosis:
- Standard detection of eggs on stool O+P

Treatment:
- Praziquantel 5–10 mg/kg PO x1 (600 mg tablets)
- (Inferior alternative) nitazoxanide 500 mg PO BID x 3 days

C. *Dipylidium caninum*

Exposure Required:
- Oral ingestion of infected adult fleas

Clinical Disease:
- Asymptomatic

Diagnosis:
- Standard detection of eggs on stool O+P

Treatment:
- Praziquantel 5–10 mg/kg PO x1 (600 mg tablets)
- (Inferior alternative) nitazoxanide 500 mg PO BID x 3 days

32. Juvenile Tapeworm Infections of Humans

A. *Echinococcus granulosus*

Exposure Required:
- Oral ingestion of embryonated eggs

Clinical Disease:
- Liver cysts, lung cysts, cysts in any organ, anaphylactic reactions with cyst rupture

Diagnosis:
- Imaging: cysts can be visualized with CT, MRI and ultrasound
- Microscopy: examination of cyst contents and cysts themselves
- Serological testing: sensitivities vary by cyst stage
- NAAT

Treatment:
- Based on Stage CE1–CE5:
    - CE1
        - < 5cm - Albendazole 400 mg PO BID
        - > 5cm - Albendazole 400 mg PO BID and puncture, aspiration injection, re-aspiration (PAIR)
    - CE3a
        - < 5cm - Albendazole 400 mg PO BID
        - > 5cm - Albendazole 400 mg PO BID and PAIR
    - CE2 - Albendazole 40 0 mg PO BID and large bore percutaneous treatment, (PAIR is contraindicated)
    - CE3b - Albendazole 400 mg PO BID and large bore percutaneous treatment, (PAIR is contraindicated)
    - CE4 & CE5 - observation with imaging every 6 months, (PAIR is contraindicated)
    - Surgery - indicated for cysts >10 cm, ruptured cysts, extra-hepatic disease, very complex cysts (many daughter cells) and cysts that have formed fistula.

B. *Echinococcus multilocularis*

Exposure Required:
- Oral ingestion of embryonated eggs

Clinical Disease:
- Proliferative membranes primarily in the liver leading to hepatic failure, abdominal pain, weight loss, fatigue

Diagnosis:
- Imaging - lesions can be visualized with CT, MRI and ultrasound
- Microscopy - histology of directed biopsy specimens
- Serological testing - sensitive and specific enough to distinguish from *E. granulosus*
- NAAT

Treatment:
- Surgery is the primary approach when possible
- Albendazole 400 mg PO BID suggested minimum of 2 years but indefinitely if not amenable to surgery

C. *Mesocestoides* spp.

Exposure Required:
- Oral ingestion of infective larvae in under cooked bird, snake, lizard, amphibian or mammalian carnivore

Clinical Disease:
- Mild abdominal discomfort, nausea, diarrhea, vomiting

Diagnosis:
- Detection of eggs on stool O+P

Treatment:
- Praziquantel 5–10 mg/kg PO x1 (600 mg tablets)
- (Inferior alternative) nitazoxanide 500 mg PO BID x 3 days

D. *Spirometra* spp.

Exposure Required:
- Oral ingestion of infective larvae in undercooked meat or exposure to larvae from poultice that then invade through wound or mucous membrane

Clinical Disease:
- Asymptomatic, orbital edema, neurological complications

Diagnosis:
- Identification of the parasite after removal or biopsy

Treatment:
- Primarily Surgical Management

E. *Taenia* spp. (other than *T. saginata* and *T. solium*)

Exposure Required:
- Oral ingestion of embryonated eggs

Clinical Disease:
- Mass effect in organ invaded, may invade CNS (brain, eyes, spinal cord)

Diagnosis:
- Identification of the parasite after removal or biopsy

Treatment:
- Primarily surgical management

33. The Schistosomes
Schistosoma mansoni
Schistosoma japonicum
Schistosoma haematobium
Schistosoma mekongi
Schistosoma intercalatum

Exposure Required:
- Infective cercariae enter skin (usually through a hair follicle)

Clinical Disease:
- **Acute** – 'Katayama fever' hepatomegaly, splenomegaly, lymphadenopathy, fever, myalgias, cough, headache, eosinophilia
- **Chronic** – abdominal pain, diarrhea, hepatomegaly, splenomegaly, hematuria, vaginal symptoms in female genital schistosomiasis (FGS), CNS - (focal transverse myelitis, encephalitis)

Diagnosis:
- Microscopy: detection of schistosome eggs in stool or urine. Detection of eggs in an unfixed rectal snip/biopsy
- Antigen detection: two schistosome glycoprotein antigens known as CCA and CAA circulate in the bloodstream of acutely infected patients and can be detected with certain assays
- Serology: antibodies develop 6–12 weeks after exposure and tend to become positive before eggs are evident in urine or stool. (ELISA, indirect hemagglutination assay (IHA), radioimmunoassay, complement fixation, Western blot)
- Imaging: portable ultrasound imaging has been shown to be clinically useful in the diagnosis of schistosomiasis

Treatment:
Detection of viable eggs 6 weeks after treatment warrants retreatment
- **Acute Infection**
    - Prednisone 40 mg PO Q-day x 5 days
    - Praziquantel 20 mg/kg PO TID x 1 day (6 weeks after exposure and when acute symptoms have resolved) then repeated 6 weeks later (600 mg tablets)
- **Chronic Infection**
    - Praziquantel 20 mg/kg PO TID x 1 day (8 weeks after exposure and when acute symptoms have resolved) (600 mg tablets)
- **CNS Schistosomiasis**
    - Prednisone 1mg/kg PO Q-day started immediately with duration based on response and clinical course

34. *Clonorchis sinensis* and *Opisthorchis* spp.

Exposure Required:
- Oral ingestion of raw or undercooked freshwater fish containing metacercariae

Clinical Disease:
- Asymptomatic, right upper quadrant abdominal pain, nausea, diarrhea, headache, hepatomegaly, eosinophilia

Diagnosis:
- Microscopy - after 4 weeks eggs will be released into feces. The sensitivity can be improved with NAAT (PCR and loop-mediated isothermal amplification ([LAMP])
- Endoscopy - endoscopic retrograde cholangiopancreatography (ERCP) may allow visualization of flukes
- Serology - ELISA with confirmatory Western blot is available
- Imaging - the presence of flukes in the biliary tract may also be observed using ultrasound, CT, MRI and cholangiography

Treatment:
- **Antiparasitics**
  - Praziquantel 25 mg/kg PO TID x 2 days or praziquantel 40 mg/kg PO x1 for light infections (600 mg tablets)
  - Albendazole 10 mg/kg PO Q-day x 7 days
  - Mebendazole 30 mg/kg PO Q-day x 30 days
- **Mechanical Interventions**
  - Surgery, biliary drainage and broad-spectrum antibiotics may be required in certain cases

35. *Fasciola hepatica*

Exposure Required:
- Oral ingestion of metacercariae on watercress or other littoral plants

Clinical Disease:
- Early phase – fever, right upper quadrant abdominal pain, malaise, headache, eosinophilia
- Chronic – dull right upper quadrant pain, biliary obstruction

Diagnosis:
- Serology - serological tests become positive early in disease during migration through the liver parenchyma
- Antigen tests - available with high sensitivity and specificity
- Microscopy - after 4 months eggs will start to be released into feces
- Endoscopy - endoscopic retrograde cholangiopancreatography (ERCP) may allow visualization of flukes
- Imaging - the presence of linear migratory tracts and adult flukes may also be observed using ultrasound, CT, MRI and cholangiography

Treatment:
In the United States Triclabendazole can be obtained through the CDC.
- Triclabendazole 10 mg/kg PO x1 and then in severe infections may be repeated 12–24 hrs after the first dose. Successfully treated patients will develop negative serologies 6–12 months after clearing their parasites.
- (Inferior alternative) Nitazoxanide 500 mg PO BID for 7 days

36. *Paragonimus westermani / P. kellicotti*

Exposure Required:
- Oral ingestion of metacercariae on raw or undercooked crab or crustaceans

Clinical Disease:
- Acute - asymptomatic, diarrhea, fever, chest pain, fatigue, urticaria, epigastric pain, eosinophilia
- Late – fever, chills, cough, dyspnea, blood tinged sputum, hemoptysis, pulmonary infiltrates, pulmonary lesions, CNS-more common with *P. kellicotti*

Diagnosis:
- Serology - serological tests are important in early disease before egg production occurs which can take 8–12 weeks
- Microscopy - late-stage disease is diagnosed by microscopic identification of eggs in the sputum, bronchoalveolar lavage fluid, and, more rarely, in stool
- Imaging - ultrasound, X-ray examinations, CT, MRI and fluorodeoxyglucose-positron emission tomography (FDG-PET)

Treatment:
- Praziquantel 25 mg/kg PO TID for 3 days (600 mg tablets)
- Triclabendazole 10 mg/kg PO x1

37. Other Trematodes of Medical Importance

A. *Fasciolopsis buski*

Exposure Required:
- Oral ingestion of metacercariae on husks of seeds of littoral plants such as water chestnuts

Clinical Disease:
- Asymptomatic, diarrhea, vomiting, nausea, fever, intestinal hemorrhage, abdominal pain, eosinophilia

Diagnosis:
- Microscopy - identification of eggs or flukes in stool or vomit

Treatment:
- Praziquantel 25 mg/kg PO TID x 1 day (600 mg tablets)

B. *Echinostoma* spp.

Exposure Required:
- Oral ingestion of metacercariae from ingesting various species of snails, tadpoles, or freshwater fish

Clinical Disease:
- Diarrhea, nausea, vomiting, abdominal pain, fever

Diagnosis:
- Microscopy - identification of eggs in stool or in some cases flukes recovered from endoscopy

Treatment:
- Praziquantel 25 mg/kg PO x 1 day (600 mg tablets)

C. *Heterophyes heterophyes/Metagonimus yokogawai*

Exposure Required:
- Oral ingestion of metacercariae from ingesting certain freshwater fish

Clinical Disease:
- Epigastric pain, fatigue, diarrhea, weight loss, malaise, belching, nausea, headache, vomiting

Diagnosis:
- Microscopy - identification of eggs in stool
- NAAT – only available in research settings

Treatment:
- Praziquantel 25 mg/kg PO TID x 1 day (600 mg tablets)

D. *Nanophyetus salmincola*

Exposure Required:
- Ingestion of raw or undercooked salmon containing metacercariae

Clinical Disease:
- Diarrhea, nausea, vomiting, anorexia, eosinophilia

Diagnosis:
- Microscopy: identification of eggs in stool

Treatment:
- Praziquantel 25 mg/kg PO TID x 1 day (600 mg tablets)
- Niclosamide 2 g PO x1 (not commercially available in the United States)

38. The Insects

A. Myiasis-Causing Flies: Calliphoridae, Cuterebridae, and Sarcophagidae

Exposure Required:
- Larvae penetrate intact skin or wounds

Clinical Disease:
- Abscess like swellings with openings, maggots visible in wounds

Diagnosis:
- Visualization of living or dead maggots, but suggested by abscess like lesions with small central opening

Treatment:
- Surgical removal is the primary treatment
- Alternatively, if the opening is blocked with a substance such as petroleum jelly, that blocks access to oxygen, they can be forced to crawl to the surface and be removed

B. Anaplura: Sucking Lice

Exposure Required:
- Direct contact with an infected individual for hair lice / physical contact and clothing for body lice

Clinical Disease:
- Pruritis

Diagnosis:
- Visualization of lice or eggs in the hair or seams of garments. The wet combing technique increases sensitivity for detection of lice attached to hair.

Treatment:
- **For body lice:**
    - Manual removal of lice using the wet combing technique can be performed
    - Topical application of pediculicides (for age >2 months of age - permethrin (1%) cream rinse leave on hair for 10 minutes, rinse off and repeat 9 days later, > 6 months of age benzyl alcohol (5%) lotion leave on hair for 10 minutes, rinse off and repeat 7 days later, > 6 months of age ivermectin (0.5%) topical lotion leave on hair for 10 minutes, rinse off, > 2 years of age pyrethrins (0.33%) with piperonyl butoxide (4%) lotion apply to dry hair and leave on hair for 10 minutes, rinse off and repeat 9 days later.
    - (Alternative) > 6 years of age – malathion (0.5%) lotion leave on hair for 8–12 hrs then wash off, may repeat in 9 days
    - Oral treatment with ivermectin 200–400 mcg/kg PO x1 (3 mg tablets so ~5–6 tablets for a 70 kg adult) with a second treatment on day 8 if live lice detected
- **For body lice:**
    - Thoroughly bathe patient and wash clothing in heated water >149 ° F, occasionally topical therapy with permethrin (5%) cream to entire body and left on for 8–10 hrs. Low potency topical steroids may be used for symptomatic relief.
    - Oral treatment with ivermectin 200–400 mcg/kg PO x1 may have a transient impact on body lice infestation
- **For pubic lice:**
    - Manual removal of lice using the wet combing technique can be performed
    - Topical application of pediculicides (for age >2 months of age – permethrin (1%) cream rinse, leave on affected areas for 10 minutes, pyrethrins (0.33%) with piperonyl butoxide (4%) lotion apply to affected areas and leave on hair for 10 minutes
    - Oral treatment with ivermectin 250 mcg/kg PO x1 (3mg tablets so ~5–6 tablets for a 70 kg adult) repeated 1–2 weeks later

39. The Arachnids

A. Ticks

Exposure Required:
- Exposure to ticks

Clinical Disease:
- Various manifestations for different tick-borne diseases, imbedded tick

Diagnosis:
- Visualization of the tick

Treatment:
- Gently but firmly pulling the tick away from its point of attachment so the entire tick, including its mouthparts, is removed. It is recommended that chemical means be avoided and burning or smothering ticks is not attempted.

B. Scabies: *Sarcoptes scabiei*

Exposure Required:
- Direct contact with an infected individual

Clinical Disease:
- Itching, skin rash

Diagnosis:
- Skin scraping and microscopic identification of scabies mites, eggs or feces. Dermoscopy can be helpful to visualize burrows, mites and identification of 'delta wing' sign and also to direct scrapings.

Treatment:
- Topical application of permethrin (1%) cream leave on entire body including under the nails for 8–14 hrs, rinse off and repeat 1–2 weeks later if needed, 30 g typically required to cover entire body
- Oral treatment with ivermectin 200 mcg/kg PO x1 (3mg tablets so ~5 tablets for a 70 kg adult) with a second treatment on day 8 if live lice detected

Important note: A clinician experienced in the treatment of these diseases should guide all diagnostic modality and treatment selections. This appendix serves as a quick reference guide, but we recommend review of this material with sources of updated treatment and diagnosis such as the CDC before making diagnostic or treatment decisions. We also recommend that exact dosing, side effects, drug interactions and consideration of patient allergies be verified and considered.

Exposures

Exposure/Infection	
Oral (typically contaminated food or water)	Amoebiasis, Angiostrongyliasis, Anisakiasis, Ascariasis Balantidiasis, Baylisascariasis, Blastocystosis Clonorchiasis, Cryptosporidiosis, Cyclosporiasis, Cysticercosis, Cystoisosporiasis Dientamoebiasis, Diphyllobothriasis, Dracunculiasis Echinococcosis Fascioliasis Giardiasis, Gnathostomiasis Hepatic capillariasis Intestinal capillariasis Mesocestoidiasis Oesophagostomiasis Paragonimiasis, Pin worms Sparganosis Taeniasis-meat, Ternidensiasis, Toxoplasmosis, Trichinellosis, Trichuriasis VLM/OLM
Vector (flies, mosquitos, insect feces, ticks, midges)	African Trypanosomiasis (Tsetse fly), American Trypanosomiasis (Reduviid bug feces) Babesiosis (tick bite) Dirofilariasis (mosquito) Leishmaniasis (sand fly), Loiasis (deer fly), Lymphatic filariasis (mosquito) Malaria (mosquito), Mansonellosis (black flies/midges) Onchocerciasis (black fly)
Contact (mucous membranes, intact skin, wounds)	Acanthamoebiasis, American Trypanosomiasis Hookworms Larva Migrans, Lice (includes human-human contact) Myiasis Naeglariasis Scabies (includes human-human contact), Schistosomiasis, Sparganosis, Strongyloidiasis Ticks, Trichomoniasis (includes human-human contact)
Respiratory (inhalation)	Acanthamoebiasis Balamuthiasis Toxoplasmosis

Diagnostic and Laboratory Abnormalities

Diagnostics and Laboratory Abnormalities	
Anemia	Babesiosis, Hookworms, Malaria, Trichuriasis
Arrhythmias	American Trypanosomiasis, Trichinellosis
Eosinopenia	Malaria
Eosinophilia	Angiostrongyliasis, Ascariasis-migration, Clonorchiasis, Cryptosporidiosis, Dientamoebiasis, Hepatic capillariasis, Hookworm-migration, Fascioliasis, Loiasis, Lymphatic filariasis-TPE, Mansonellosis, Paragonimiasis, Schistosomiasis, Strongyloidiasis, Trichinellosis, VLM
Eosinophils in CNS	Angiostrongyliasis, Baylisascariasis, Gnathostomiasis, Schistosomiasis
Hepatomegaly	Ascariasis, Baylisascariasis, Clonorchiasis, Leishmaniasis-visceral, Schistosomiasis, Toxoplasmosis
Lesions in CNS	Amoebiasis - rare, Baylisascariasis, Cysticercosis, Toxoplasmosis, Paragonimiasis
Lesion in Liver	Amoebiasis, Echinococcosis, Fascioliasis
Lesion in Lungs	Amoebiasis – rare, Dirofilariasis, Echinococcosis, Paragonimiasis
Lesion in Spleen	Echinococcosis
Leukocytosis	Trichinellosis
Leukopenia	Malaria, Babesiosis
Liver Failure	Hepatic capillariasis

Symptoms

Abdominal Pain\GI symptoms	Giardiasis, American Trypanosomiasis, Malaria, Cryptosporidiosis, Amoebiasis, Balantidiasis, Cystoisosporiasis, Naeglariasis, Blastocystosis, Dientamoebiasis, Trichuriasis-tenesmus, Ascariasis, Strongyloidiasis, Trichinellosis, Hepatic capillariasis, Oesophagostomiasis, Ternidensiasis, Baylisascariasis, Angiostrongyliasis-costaricensis, Anisakiasis, Mesocestoidiasis, Schistosomiasis, Clonorchiasis, Fascioliasis, Paragonimiasis
Anal Irritation	Pin worms
Diarrhea	Giardiasis, Cryptosporidiosis, Amoebiasis, Balantidiasis, Cystoisosporiasis, Cyclosporiasis, Blastocystosis, Dientamoebiasis, Trichuriasis, Strongyloidiasis, Trichinellosis, Intestinal capillariasis, Anisakiasis, Mesocestoidiasis, Schistosomiasis, Paragonimiasis
Pulmonary symptoms	American Trypanosomiasis, Malaria, Toxoplasmosis, Ascariasis, Hookworms, Lymphatic filariasis-TPE, Echinococcosis, Schistosomiasis
Neurological symptoms	African Trypanosomiasis, American Trypanosomiasis, Toxoplasmosis, Naeglariasis, Acanthamoebiasis, Balamuthiasis, Trichinellosis, Loiasis, Visceral larva migrans-cognitive defects, Baylisascariasis, Angiostrongyliasis, Sparganosis, Schistosomiasis
Facial Swelling	African Trypanosomiasis, American Trypanosomiasis, Trichinellosis, Sparganosis
Fever or Chills	Leishmaniasis-visceral, American Trypanosomiasis, Malaria, Toxoplasmosis, Balantidiasis, Babesiosis, Naeglariasis, Acanthamoebiasis, Balamuthiasis, Trichinellosis, Lymphatic filariasis, Angiostrongyliasis, Anisakiasis, Schistosomiasis, Fascioliasis, Paragonimiasis
Headache	African Trypanosomiasis, Babesiosis, Naeglariasis, Acanthamoebiasis, Balamuthiasis, Angiostrongyliasis, Cysticercosis, Clonorchiasis, Fascioliasis
Lymphadenopathy	African Trypanosomiasis, Toxoplasmosis, Onchocerciasis, Hepatic capillariasis-abdominal, Mansonellosis-ozzardi
Lymphedema\Edema	American Trypanosomiasis, Lymphatic filariasis, Loiasis, Trichinellosis-bilateral periorbital edema
Malaise\Fatigue	American Trypanosomiasis, Toxoplasmosis, Balantidiasis, Babesiosis, Cystoisosporiasis, Lymphatic filariasis-TPE, Baylisascariasis, Diphyllobothriasis
Myalgia	Trichinellosis, Cysticercosis-localized, Schistosomiasis
Nodules/Swelling	Onchocerciasis, Loiasis, Mansonellosis-perstans, Gnathostomiasis, Cysticercosis
Ocular symptoms	Acanthamoebiasis, Onchocerciasis, Loiasis, Mansonellosis-perstans, Ocular larva migrans, Baylisascariasis
Pruritis	African Trypanosomiasis, Mansonellosis, Onchocerciasis
Seizures	African Trypanosomiasis, Toxoplasmosis, Cysticercosis
Skin changes\Rash	Leishmaniasis-visceral, Hookworms, Onchocerciasis, Mansonellosis, Larva Migrans
Ulcers	Leishmaniasis-cutaneous, African Trypanosomiasis, Dracunculiasis
Vaginal symptoms	Trichomoniasis, Schistosomiasis

www.ingramcontent.com/pod-product-compliance
Lightning Source LLC
Chambersburg PA
CBHW081020170526
45158CB00010B/3115